DIY
homemade
FACE MASK
STEP-BY-STEP PICTURES

Susan Holt

TABLE OF CONTENTS

Introduction:

When a person knows how to do everything himself, he does not depend on circumstances. Crafting is an enjoyable hobby. One should create things from those they already have. A mask is a general requirement for protecting one's self from the environment. So the idea to make a mask for yourself is not superfluous.

And so, if you set yourself the goal of making a mask for yourself or your loved ones, a lot of questions might spring up in your mind. You are lucky because you can get answers to all those questions in this book.

I tried to gather here a brief, but in-depth information about the masks, how they work, the pathogens they can protect you from, and how to use them. It has a detailed description of the fabrics that can be used for making a mask. This book has lessons to guide you how to make a mask for yourself!

And most importantly, to manufacture a mask you do not need any special devices, except for simple threads and needles, or some other improvised means which are discussed in this book. And you don't need any special skills, believe me, I experienced it myself, and I'm not an expert by I did it. This is easy but worth doing.

your time is essential to me, so the book contains as much as possible useful and practical information that you can take and use in order to learn how to make masks in a short time.

And so, if you want to protect yourself during the periods of exacerbation in the world. When infections are waiting for you at your doorstep so, use this book, make your own mask, stay calm and feel the charm. Yeah, obviously living in an environment full of diseases you must also consider other preventive and proper guidelines that were discussed side by side in this book.

History

Mask is protecting medical equipment. It comforts you in different situations of life. The invention and implication of masks go back to a medical emergency in the world in the 19th century, that gave birth to this useful and protective equipment. It was more often called the plague's doctor mask, which first came into the application during the bubonic breakout in Europe. It was the era of the Middle Ages. The first medical mask has glass coverings for the eye openings and a beak that contains some garlic, salts, and other herbs for medicinal purposes. These contents present created an antibacterial environment. In the 19th century, people used wool bandage as a mask that had a valve for support. This is how the use of medical masks came into existence.

Later on, the old masks were replaced with new and advance kind of masks. During those days, a widely spread disease called "Spanish flu" occurred. It took lives of about a hundred million people. Initially, cotton masks were used by people.

In the 20th century, the widespread use of disposable masks was seen. Polymeric materials that were prepared synthetically were used for making these disposable masks. They can be frequently seen today. That is how the use of masks began and evolved with time to aid the doctors, medical staff, and humanity.

Modern Era and Masks

We are living in a modern world where each day brings innovation to your life. Changes are always good as new things add up to your life. The medical mask we use today is not the same that was used in the 19th century. Gauze bandage mask was the first type of mask ever used. Gauze is a surgical material that is resistant to autoclaving. It is inexpensive material so that is why it was most commonly used. But the masks used today are somewhat different. Nowadays, the polymeric substance is used for making medical masks. They are spunbond, unlike gauze bandage masks. The modern mask has three layers. There is a filter in the middle layer of the mask. The modern mask has a specific aluminium insert that is added for the support at the nose. It keeps the mask right at its place. There are accessories attached to the mask, which include ear loops, a layer of a hydrophobic material, a screen along with a film. We can easily understand that ear loops keep the mask at its place as they hold it between ears. A layer of hydrophobic material is added to the mask. It is to resist the moisture content. Additional layers might be added to the mask to enhance its protective effect. The additional layers include a screen and a protective film. The film is to prevent the contact of biological fluids with the mask whereas the screen is specially designed to protect the formation of fog inside spectacles.

Classification of Masks

Generally, medical masks have been divided into two categories based on their use and role. There are two types of medical masks based on there use. This classification is specific for the non-woven polymeric Masks

* ★ Procedural Mask
* ★ Surgical Mask

Procedural Masks

The procedural mask can be defined as the one used for daily life purposes. An individual can make it a part of one's daily routine. Procedural Mask is often referred to as regular or every day's mask. The procedural mask consists of three layers, an inner layer and outer layer, while a middle layer consists of a filter. Procedural masks are designed by placing a filter in between two layers of fabric. There are two types of procedural masks. One is for the adults and one for children. The adult mask is 175×95 mm, whereas that used for children is 140×80 mm.

Surgical Masks

Surgical masks are used by doctors, nurses, and paramedics during surgery. Surgical masks are prepared using a non-woven fabric. Surgical Mask has four different layers. Three of them are similar to that of the procedural mask. Along with them is the fluid-resistant barrier. The fluid-resistant layer has been placed to inhibit the entrance and contact of biological fluids with skin while carrying out surgical procedures. There is a screen attached to the surgical masks to prevent the formation of fog on glasses. Surgical masks should be used in specific conditions only. They are further classified as sterile or non-sterile. Sterile masks are expensive so procedural masks as are preferred upon the surgical masks for everyday use. However, there are some cases in which we might feel the need to use a sterile mask. Operation theatres, labs, and sterilized rooms are the places where it is necessary to keep the environment sterile. It is not easy to manufacture sterile masks because of the high costs rendered during the process. So, to make our procedures economically feasible sterile masks are limited to certain vicinities and not ordinary rooms.

From What and How the Mask Protects

Coughing and sneezing bring out some contents from the body that are harmful to others. They are pathogens actually. When a person coughs, he or she pulls out the air along with droplets from the respiratory tract forcefully. Coughing is not a normal phenomenon. It does not usually place. Whenever a person's respiratory system is facing obstructions in the continuous flow of air, cough occurs. The same goes for sneezing! It is not a normal process, and the person might need to do this after being the victim of common cold, flu, or other viral diseases. During coughing and sneezing a person expels out harmful substances and mucus. Virus and bacteria may be present in the mucous. The sick person unintentionally adds infectious agents to the environment. They affect the healthy individuals So here comes the protective and beneficial effect of the mask. If the person is wearing a mask, the tiny droplets he coughs or sneezes are held within the mask. It saves the other person, the healthy one, from inhaling those viral droplets. An infectious agent can enter the body of a healthy individual if one touches the contaminated surface. But if you are wearing a mask, it serves as a barrier and protects you from becoming the innocent victim of these viruses. The masks you wear have a specific pore size, so it can only prevent and protect you from a certain size of harmful agents that might enter your body; however, too small particles can not be blocked. The virus is the smallest entity among all disease-causing agents, and the pore size of filter material placed in the mask is often ineffective, so the viral diseases are easily transmitted to the other person. However, what we are looking for is to make the possibility of transmission minimum. Masks aid in reducing the transfer of infection through coughing, sneezing, and through contact.

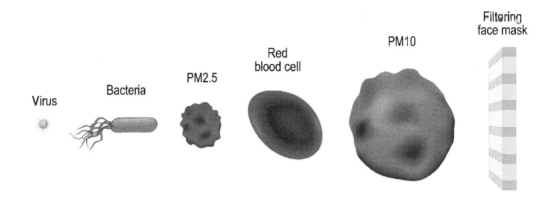

With a little bit of imperfection of masks, comes a device called a "Respirator." It is more reliable than simple masks. It fits onto the face. It fits more tightly to the face than a procedural and surgical mask. Hence, provides better filtration.

One can prevent pathogens from entering the body by taking proper care. Avoid touching the mask you are wearing so that any infectious organism might not stick to it. Wash hands often, this is because the infectious organism might have stuck on your hands, and when you touch the mask, it gains entry to your body. Frequently washing hands with soap and water removes the viral particle from your hands and creates a disinfected environment.

We can prevent the mask from being contaminated by using a disposable covering. One can wear a disposable covering over the mask which can be later. This practice creases the frequency of using the same mask often.

These are some tips that an individual can follow for the efficient use of a mask. If a person wears a mask made up of any kind of fabric and strictly follows the guidelines, he/she can limit the transmittance of infectious diseases. One must know the certain contagious disease that can transmit in the absence of a mask. These include:

- ★ Viral diseases like mumps, measles, common cold, influenza, and chickenpox. Viral diseases are better to be prevented rather than treated.
- ★ Bacterial diseases include diphtheria, meningitis, whooping cough, meningococcal, and scarlet fever. Wash your hands with soap often to remove the harmful bacteria from your skin.
- ★ Allergic diseases can be managed by the use of a mask. A person might be allergic to any inhalant or investment. Using a mask prevents its entry into the body.

What do you think about wearing a mask? Is this idea superfluous?

Prevention is better than cure. This is a common phrase which can be easily understood by everyone. It is even easier to prevent a disease rather than fighting it. Would you like to treat a disease with medicines your stomach can not tolerate, and your pocket can't bear? Or would you just like to wear a mask to alleviate your comfort further?

Infected persons add up infectious particles to the air when they cough and sneeze, so it is a good choice to save yourself from those diseases by wearing a mask. Scientists were confused about the idea of wearing a mask. Some of them said it is favourable while the rest were still looking for an authentic approach. For this purpose, they conducted several clinical trials. Public places and medical vicinities were the locations for these trials. Scientists came to know that the use of mask at public places was useful, as it saved healthy individuals by becoming a victim to airborne diseases. Masks at public places protected the respiratory organs of healthy individuals. However, the observations drawn out from the individuals at the hospital were different. Wearing a mask in a hospital didn't help much and this was because of the highly contaminated environment of hospitals. Specially designed respirators can create a difference.

World Health Organization's Recommendation About Mask!

WHO initially guides about the personal hygiene of an individual. The possibility of getting ill depends on how clean an individual lives. WHO recommends the use of medical masks to prevent airborne diseases. A mask can work in normal days but not when an infectious agent has attacked the world, for example in the case of Influenza that spreads rapidly. In the case of increased risk of catching the disease like chronic respiratory tract infections, or tuberculosis, etc., WHO recommends wearing a respirator.

Rules to Wear a Mask

There are certain rules to follow for wearing a mask for better safety and protection.

Mask is not an ornamental addition to enhance your outlook, but it is a device that you are using for protection from the outside environment and its contaminants. People often don't follow the guidelines and then, that they are not getting the required results. For anything that you aim to get, first follow the rules strictly. A mask can enhance your safety. Wear a mask properly, that is according to guidelines otherwise you will not get expected results. It is obligatory to wash your hands before wearing a mask and after removing it.

There is another question that revolves around one's mind. Well! It depends upon the need. The time period varies from 2-6 hours. In the case of the epidemic and then being in a hospital, never wear a mask for more than two hours. This is because the hospital's environment has more infectious agents as compared to the environment outside. The mask you are wearing is contaminated easier and sooner. Apart from this, if you are wearing a mask for protection from smoke or smog, then it is wearable for 6 hours. The stated details give you a clear picture of how the external environment affects the duration of wearing a mask.

★ If the mask you are wearing is damaged or becomes dirty, immediately replace it with another mask. Don't forget to wash your hands after putting off and before wearing a new mask. Then dispose of the dirty or damaged mask by putting it in a plastic wrap. You need to wash your hands again.

★ Do not eat or drink while wearing a mask. Do not even try this by dragging the mask aside because this would badly influence the safety that is expected from the mask. Eating and drinking by setting the mask aside is a poor practice.

★ Always wear a mask in public places. It can protect you from infections that an unknown person can transmit you.

★ Never touch the mask while you are wearing it.

★ Do not wear a damp or wet mask. Change it whenever it gets wet. This is because pathogens might find the damp atmosphere favourable and could enter your body easily.

★ The mask you are wearing should highly fit onto your face covering nose, mouth, and chin. Otherwise, unfiltered air will enter from the spaces left open bringing infectious agents along with it.

★ When you are removing a mask, use its earloops for removal and do not pull it off by grasping it completely with your hand.

★ Never use the same mask you have already used.

★ Do not put off a bandage from a mask and place it again otherwise you will aid the contamination process.

★ Wash your hands with soap after removing a mask.

★ The mask you are wearing should be tight enough to provide a proper safety but it should not be so right to harm your skin.

★ Bandages can be used with a mask to use the same mask for a longer duration. For this, you have to remove the bandages after every four hours, wash them with detergent, dry, and iron them.

Warning: It is not about wearing a mask only

Mask is indeed a protecting device. It enhances your safety but it is not enough alone if other measures for self-hygiene are not taken. There is a dire need to wear a medical mask in public gathering rather than wearing it at lonely places.

You are less likely to catch a disease while walking alone in a street in contrast to walking in a public place. It is agreed that wearing a mask reduces the risk of getting infected by a viral particle through someone's coughing or sneezing, but prior to this is personal hygiene and social distancing. Self-hygiene is not only important crucial to one's life. A person maintaining good personal hygiene can prevent disease better. When a person remains neat and clean, eats healthy, stays hydrated, keeps his surroundings clean and green, then he is living optimum health. His immune system is boosted. And here if a mask adds up, this would be a plus point to his defensive measures. But if a person does not live hygienically, eats unhealthily, breathes polluted, then wearing a mask won't help him much. One must understand the importance of social distancing as it may save a healthy individual from falling prey to the illnesses, he hasn't thought of having. Social distancing can be defined as maintaining a physical distance from one another. It is a good practice to stop the spread of diseases. There are three points which a person should follow to adopt social distancing. For this you need

- ★ Stay 6 feet away from each other
- ★ Do not gather at public places
- ★ Avoid gatherings

Choice of Fabric for Mask

When it comes to making a mask for yourself, the first thing that comes to mind is the choice of fabric. What should be the mask made up of? From where would I get it? The answer to these questions will ease your difficulty. Just keep in mind that the fabric you are using for making a mask must be holistic and easily breathable. There must be no stains on it, which means you need a clean and washed piece of cloth for it. We can make a mask out of any old cotton bed sheet or a pillowcase. Any cotton curtain removed from the window or your old t-shirt. All these materials can be used for making a mask. You can even make your own clothes for it. There are different materials available in the market which we can buy for making a mask for ourselves.

Polyester: It is a commercially used fabric that is not woven actually. The material has lesser pores and pore size than ordinary fabric. It is a synthetic material. It is spun-bold amazingly that the holes between the fabric become maximally small. The material is hygienic to use. It gives good filtration. The particles larger than the pore size settle on it.

Satin: Satin is mostly used in summer clothing. It allows good air ventilation across it so it is a good choice for making masks. Generally, it is used in making beddings, baby clothes and T-shirts. It is a soft material so easy to wear and does not bother one's skin. Its fibres are resistant to washing and can withstand the effect of high temperature.

Flannel: Flannel is a woven fabric. There are different varieties of flannel depending upon softness. Due to its soft texture, it is considered skin-friendly. It is engrossed with a pattern that does not fade away by washing, so it is a good choice for making masks. Flannel masks can be washed and reused hence economical. Flannel was initially made using wool but nowadays it is prepared synthetically.

Viscose: This kind of fabric acquires a look like silk, wool, or linen. It is made up of cellulose and then introduced with an additive. Viscose is commonly used in dressings. It has a good filtration ability so we can consider viscose as a good choice for making masks. It allows a steady airflow creating a ventilated environment. However, masks made up of viscose should not be washed frequently as this fabric loses shape by washing.

Linen: Linen is a fabric that is made using flax fibres. During the process of preparing fibre out of flax, knots are woven within the fibre. It gives the material a good strength. The material is resistant to allergenic substances so is often used for making a mask. It dries quickly so linen masks can be frequently washed.

Calico: A suitable fabric for making masks. It is used frequently for this purpose. Calico has thicker fibres, as compared to other fabrics. It has a characteristic weave pattern that makes it different from others. It is woven in a criss-cross pattern. This pattern makes it compact such that it gives efficient filtration. The effective filtration prevents infectious agents from entering the respiratory tract or oral cavity of humans.

Knitwear: It is a soft fabric that is commonly used. It does not harm skin so the masks made of knitwear can be worn for longer durations. Sometimes people often put an additional bandage on the mask for better protection. The bandage must be placed skilfully on the mask to prevent the formation of pointed edge that often appears.

Chintz: Chintz is actually a cotton material that is inexpensive. It is woven compactly that the high density of fibres in the fabric makes it soft to touch. Chintz bandages are cheap to buy. It does not cost you much even if you buy the cloth and then stitch a mask from it. Chintz consists of attractive designs and beautiful patterns, and one can create colourful surroundings for themselves. Chintz mask would be comfortable to wear and at the same time give you the ease of breathing.

So many options! But what's the best?

When it was difficult to decide which material should be used for making a mask, scientists worked on it. Researchers at the University of California tested different materials. The materials were tested by bombarding them with Bacteriophage MS Viruses of 0.023 microns and Bacillus atrophaeus, which ranges in size from 0.93 to 1.25 microns. Various household materials were also tested by bombarding them with similar species. At the same time, the surgical mask was tested in a similar manner and the results were compared. Researchers found that pure cotton was able to filter 69% of particles. Kitchen towels blocked 83% of particles, whereas filters for vacuum cleaners stopped 95% of particles. However, this was closest to the efficacy of surgical masks, which is 97%. Though kitchen towels and vacuum cleaners gave better filtration than pure cotton scientists declared pure cotton as the most suitable material for making a mask and this was because it allowed the users to breathe easily. It was not easy to breathe while wearing masks made up of other materials.

Double-Layered Masks

After manufacturing the protective medical masks, scientists looked for innovations in the field of masks, which could bring more comfort into the life of humans. Scientists thought that if they would double the layer of fabric used in a mask, it would give better filtration and safety. Generally, to increase the defense we can strengthen barriers. This restricts the pressure outside! The researchers found the experiment fruitful. The double-layered mask gave better protection than the single-layered mask. The materials examined included pillowcase, t-shirts, and towels. Pillowcase layers, when doubled, showed a 1% increase inefficiency. T-shirts gave 2% improved performance whereas the towels stood up with 14% improved results.

The Significance of Ease of Breathing in a Mask

Breathing is crucial to life, so it should never be risked. It is not only about wearing a mask to protect yourself from harmful agents of the environment but at the same, the focus is on breathing freely. The fabric that you chose for making a mask must allow ease of breathing. This would keep you comfortable otherwise, it would just be a headache to wear the mask rather than relief.

Whether you are making a mask for yourself at home or some scientists are designing it for the first time, comfortable breathing is the primary goal. Whenever you make a mask for yourself, chose a fabric with good filtration and ventilation at the same time. The researchers who designed the mask looked for ease of breathing in it compared to surgical masks. Scientists tested different fabrics to know which gave the best breathing comfort. For this, they studied the pressure difference of air on both sides of the fabric. It was found by the scientists that kitchen towel and vacuum cleaner filters are most efficient in filtering anonymous particles; however, it is really hard to breathe through them. Whenever you will use more than a single layer of fabric to make a mask, the difficulty to breath will eventually increase. Cotton is considered a good martial for making masks because air ventilation is easiest through it.

This is the reason researchers considered T-shirts and Pillowcase cottons the best material for making a mask. It filters 50% of particles that range in size of 0 2 microns and a person can breathe comfortably at the same time.

How to Make Your Mask Bacteria Resistant

We can improve the protection from bacteria by applying certain essential oils inside the layers of the mask. Essential oils have antimicrobial properties, antiseptic, and anti-inflammatory properties. Essential oils can boost up your immune system and can save you in many situations that due to any unwanted conditions like cold weather, polluted air, allergens etc. Let's have a look at the oils that can be used to give antibacterial properties to a mask. The process is easy as you just have to apply a thin layer of oil in the mask and that's all.

Eucalyptus Oil: Eucalyptus oil has the ability to treat cough and cold so it used frequently during winters. It has a great ability to resist bacteria so you can add a layer of eucalyptus oil to your mask.

Mint Oil: Mint oil has antibacterial action. It is also used as a flavouring agent. You can apply a layer of mint oil to your mask to add some antimicrobial action to it.

Tea tree oil: Tea tree oil has been used for decades to treat respiratory diseases. It has a vibrant anti-inflammatory action. It can resist bacteria up to a great extent so it can be applied in the mask.

Juniper Oil: Juniper Oil is an effective antimicrobial agent and also has anti-inflammatory activity. It helps to treat cough and shortness of breath. When it is applied in the mask, it adds antimicrobial properties to it. Whenever a pathogen comes in contact with the mask, due to antimicrobial action of juniper oil, it is retained outside the mask and can't enter your body.

Carnation Oil: It is a powerful antiviral agent. It also has antibacterial action at the same time. Carnation oil can be applied to the mask to increase the defense it provides you against pathogens. Carnation oil has been used frequently to layer masks.

Myrtle Oil: It is highly helpful in getting rid of runny nose and cough. It has good antimicrobial properties so that is why myrtle oil when applied to your mask, makes it microbes resistant. Myrtle oil strongly blocks viral and bacterial entities outside the mask.

Essential Oils From Citrus Fruits: Oils that are obtained from oranges and lemons have excellent antiviral and antibacterial properties. These oils are often mixed with other oils to show maximal efficacy. One can apply them alone or mixed with any other essential oil to the mask to give you better protection.

Point to Focus!

Essential oils aren't compatible with everybody's needs. They may provoke an allergic reaction in certain individuals. Some individuals might be intolerant to these oils because of the high concentration. They are highly concentrated oils so one must take care that they do not show adverse effects.

Some Methods to Make Your Own Masks

Method 1

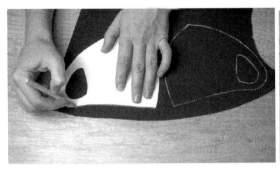 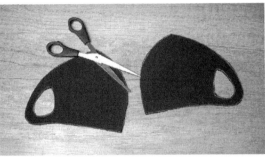

1) Encircle the stencils shown in the figure. Stencils must be encircled as each others reflection which means a mirror image to each other.

2) Cut the fabric by using a scissor.

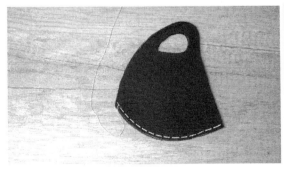 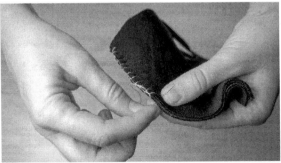

3) Fold the parts of fabric such that they both are placed above each other and stitch them on the outside, as shown in the picture

Method 2

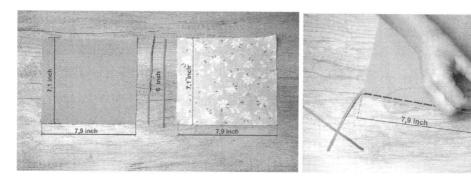

1) Cut 2 pieces of fabric 7,1x7,9 inch. This rectangular piece has two dimensions. The side with a length of 7,1 inch will stand for earloops while the 7,9 inch side will cover nose and chin.

2) Fold the fabric with the front side inward. Sweep the side with 7,9 inch.

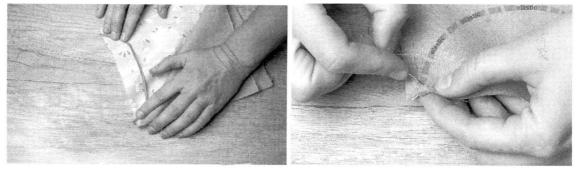

3) Sweep the side with 7,1 inch. Fix an earloop with the help of gum on the beginning of this line. Fix the other end of earloop at the end of 7,1 inch line.

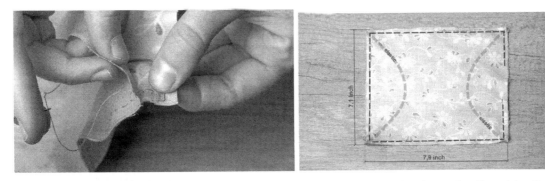

4) Sweep the other side of 7,1 inch in a similar way by placing elastic at both ends of this line.

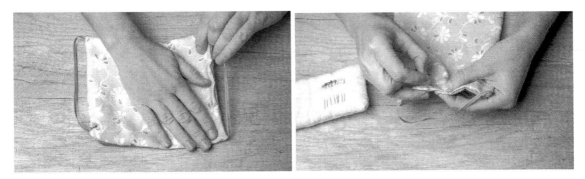

5) Iron all the edges of the mask so that everything aligns in place.

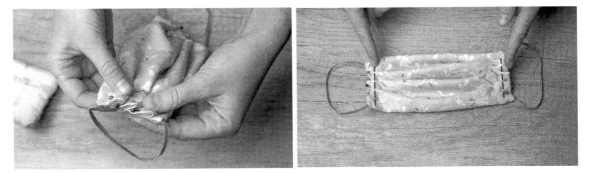

6) Make three clamps with needles on each side of the dressing

7) Sew the resulting folds from two sides, and that's it, the mask is ready

Method 3

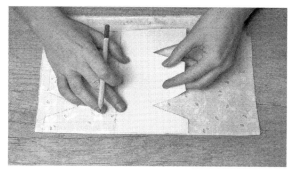 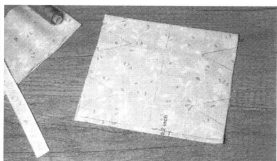

1) Fold the fabric in half such that it faces inward. Encircle the template twice such that both of these parts are a mirror image to each other.

2) Cut the resulting rectangle along the lines, only leave 0.2 inch from the bottom

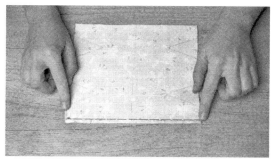 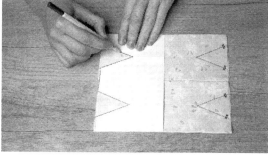

3) Sweep this side as shown in the picture.

4) Smooth the seam and twist the part. Move the seam to the middle of the part and smooth it with an iron

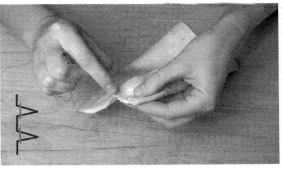 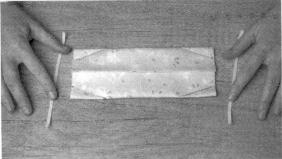

5) With the help of a stencil mark the details for the front side of the mask.

6) Sew the grooves as shown in the picture

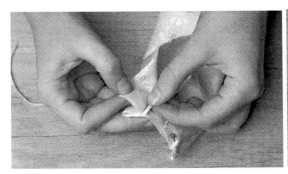 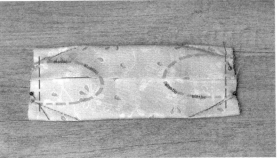

7) Take the gum, and stick their tips near the darts with needles so that the gum reaches inside of the mask. Repeat the process for the other side.

8) Sew stitches as shown in the picture, paying particular attention to those places where the ends of the elastic band are held so that they hold tight.

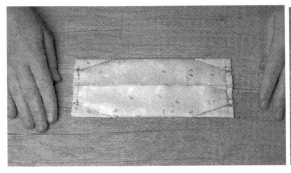 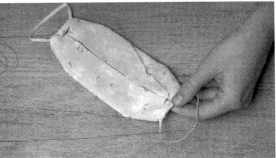

9) Iron the mask.

10) Stitch for accurate settlements.

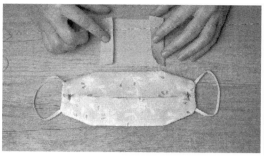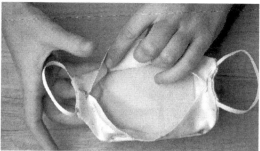

11) Cut the filter pocket as shown in the picture.

12) Insert the pocket inside the mask.

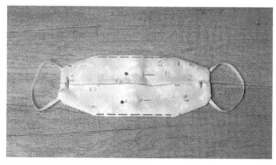

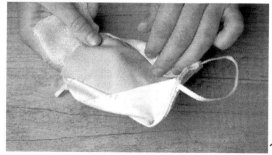13) Secure with necdles. Make two lines above and below, as shown in the picture.

14) Iron the mask, and you can insert a few layers of gauze into the pocket for comfortable breathing.

Method 4

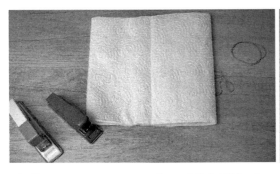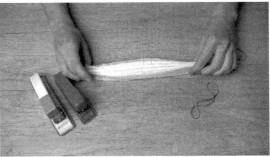

1) Take a paper towel and fold it in two layers, so that you get a square.

2) Make an "accordion" of paper and fix it on both sides with a stapler

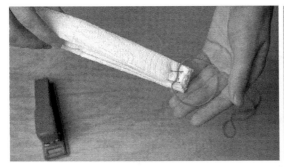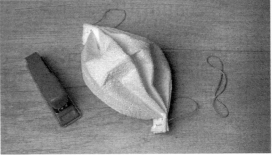

3) Also, attach a stationery eraser with a stapler to use them as ear loops

Method 5

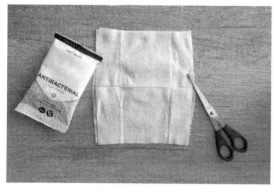 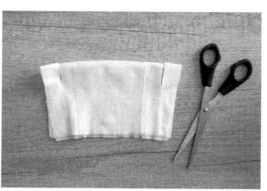

1) Take 2-4 cloth wet wipes from the package.

2) Fold them one on top of the other

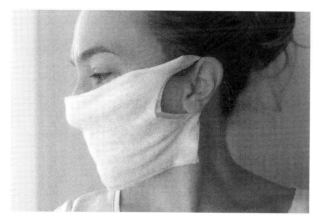

3) Make scissors cuts for the ears

4) The dressing is ready

Mask patterns for method 1 and method 3 for adults and children

For e-books download patterns from the link

https://bonusforyou.wixsite.com/mask

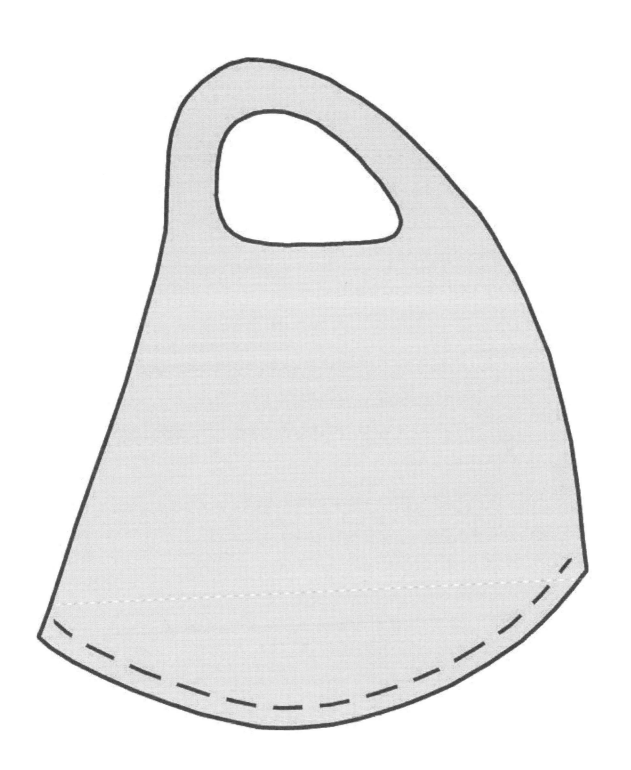

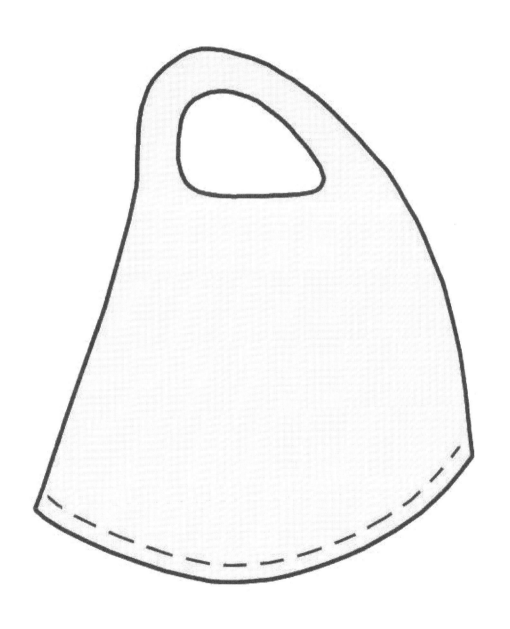

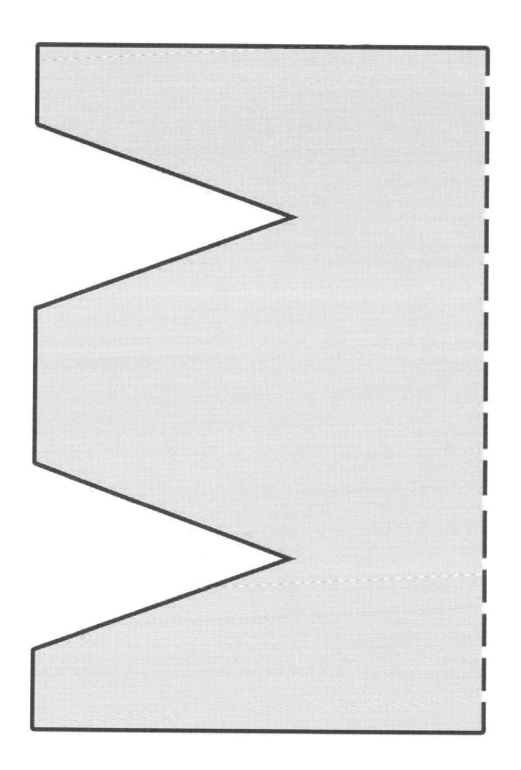

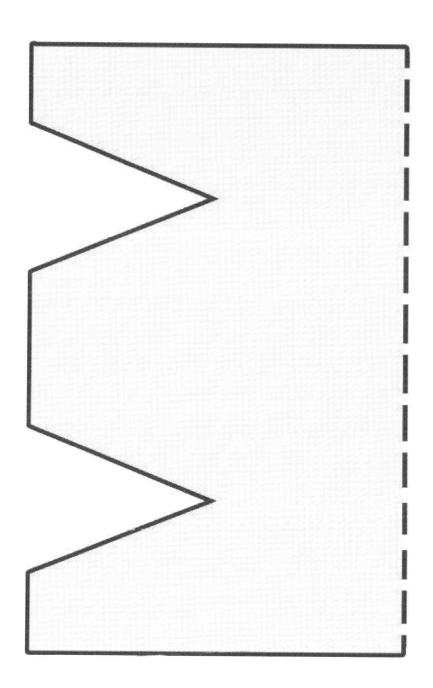

Conclusion:

Therefore, you learned about what masks are, how they can help you, and how they can be made. I hope you liked some of the lessons that you will try soon. Moreover, you have everything you need for this.

Of course, I would like you never to need this information, and that everyone in our world would always be healthy, but whoever is warned is armed, so now we can meet some life surprises calmly.

Printed in Great Britain
by Amazon

44271849R00027